What the labels won't tell you

A CONSUMER GUIDE TO HERBAL SUPPLEMENTS

What the labels won't tell you

LOGAN CHAMBERLAIN, PH.D.

INTERWEAVE PRESS

The information presented in this book is for educational purposes and should not be used as a substitute for advice from a qualified health-care practitioner. Dosage and usage information is provided as general guidelines. Some medicinal herbs may cause allergic reactions in susceptible individuals and others may not be right to use for particular health conditions.

Cover design, Bren Frisch
Cover Photography, Steven Foster

Text copyright 1998, Interweave Press, Inc.
Cover photography copyright 1998, Steven Foster

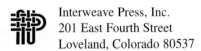 Interweave Press, Inc.
201 East Fourth Street
Loveland, Colorado 80537

Printed in the United States of America

Library of Congress Cataloging-in-Publication Date

Chamberlain, Logan, 1948–
    What the labels won't tell you: a consumer's guide to medicinal
herbs / Logan Chamberlain.
        p.   cm.
    Includes bibliographical references and index.
    ISBN 1–883010–49–7
    1. Herbs—Therapeutic use. I. Title.
RM666.H33C5141998
615'.321—dc21   98–8457
                                                                      CIP

First printing: IWP—10M: 698:UG

This book is dedicated to all of you who are looking for better ways to stay healthy using alternatives to conventional medical care.

FOREWORD

Decoding the labels. Deciding which form of supplement to use. Using herbs to stay well and avoid serious problems. These subjects and many more are covered in this much-needed book. Dr. Logan Chamberlain has brought all his resources to bear on the questions that plague consumers in their search for the most effective herbal products.

In a time when government regulations prevent manufacturers from providing their customers with the best and most complete product information, *What the Labels Won't Tell You* offers thoughtful guidance.

You'll find special sections on herbs for women and herbs for men, as well as cautions to observe when self-medicating.

I especially enjoyed the chapter on up-and-coming herbs. It's encouraging to know that we in the United States are becoming aware of such time-honored herbal remedies from our own back yard and around the world as black cohosh, horse chestnut, St. John's wort, kava kava, turmeric, and reishi.

What the Labels Won't Tell You will give you the information you need to guide you intelligently through the world of herbal supplements for your and your family's better health.

It will take a prominent place in my library, and I hope it will do the same in yours.

Dr. Earl Mindell
Author of *The Herb Bible, The Vitamin Bible, The Supplement Bible,* and *Prescription Alternatives.*

ACKNOWLEDGEMENTS

I want to thank all the people who helped me create this book. Without their considerable efforts, it would not have been possible. Thanks to Mike Corrigan and Monika Mitchell from the herb industry for their great product information. Special appreciation to Steven Foster, my herb guru and technical editor, for all his help and insights and Jim Duke for important input. Thanks to Earl Mindell for his inspiration and knowledge. Thank you to the Interweave Press team for all their efforts—especially to Stephen Beal for his wordsmithing and copy editing, and Dean Howes for his design work. Thanks to Jan Knight for supplying some vital information at the eleventh hour, to Gail Jones for her help with special projects and to Nancy Disney, who kept everything moving. And very special thanks to Linda Ligon, my partner, teacher, editor, and friend, who made this all possible.

I also want to thank my family, Susan, Lora, Logan III, and my mother, Frances, for all their support and understanding during this long but rewarding process.

TABLES AND ILLUSTRATIONS

CONTENTS

Introduction: LIVING WITH HERBS

I became interested in herbal medicine about twelve years ago. I was having some health problems—poor digestion, maybe even an ulcer—and I didn't feel very good about the course of treatment my doctor was recommending. My problems led me to seek a more traditional approach.

At that time there wasn't much popular literature on the subject of herbal medicine, but I found a book published in Europe that discussed how to use herbs for better health. It was full of testimonials that sounded believable, and I searched it for remedies that fit my gastric problems. A recipe for Swedish bitters sounded easy to make and possibly helpful, so I ordered the herbs and made a tincture from them. The results were immediate and impressive, and I was hooked on learning more about these gifts that nature provides for maintaining and improving our health.

Since then, I've lowered my blood pressure with daily doses of garlic, strengthened and regulated my heart with hawthorn, warded off many a cold with echinacea and goldenseal, cured a chronic gum abscess with a special herbal mouth tonic, and even taken a wart off my dog's lip with bloodroot. I've learned a lot by reading and asking questions, and by simple trial and error. And with every passing day I'm more convinced that herbs truly can help us stay healthy safely and naturally.

It's not easy

There's a lot of confusion on the subject of herbal medicine. We're fortunate to have so many herbal products in our pharmacies and health-food stores—the number grows daily—but we're unfortunate not to have easy access to information that will help us make the right choices. Which herb is best, say, for a sinus infection? Federal laws won't allow manufacturers to provide

> Federal laws won't allow manufacturers to provide straightforward dosage/benefit statements on their product labels.

straightforward dosage/benefit statements on their product labels, so you have to somehow figure out what to do yourself. Once you determine the herb you need, should you use capsules or tablets, liquid tinctures or extracts, or a tea? Should you look for the herb by itself, or in combination with other herbs? How much should you take, and for how long? Is there any danger in taking herbs with other medications? Is one brand or herbal preparation better than another?

These are important questions, and unless you have a trained herbalist whom you trust and depend on for advice, there's no single, easy source of information to help you make the best choices. That's why I decided to write this book. It will educate you to understand the world of herbal supplements well enough to make informed choices.

An herb is any plant or plant part that provides medical or health benefits.

What's an herb?

The term "herb" has a lot of different meanings, depending on who's using it. For instance, to a botanist an herb is any plant with soft stems that dies back every year. To a cook, it's any plant that gives special flavor to a dish. For the sake of this book I'm going to avoid any confusion by going back to an old, old meaning of the word and saying that, for our purposes, an herb is **any plant or plant part that provides medical or health benefits**.

This definition includes literally thousands of known plants from all over the world, many of which you'll probably never encounter or hear of. So I'm going to focus on the herbs that you're most likely to see discussed in current books and magazines, and displayed on the shelves at your pharmacy or health-food store. These plants have a long history of medicinal use, and in many cases, scientific and clinical studies that attest to their benefits. The list of such plants will grow as more research is done on the traditional medical practices of cultures in other parts of the world.

What parts of herbs are used for medicine?

Roots, leaves, flowers, berries, seeds—the parts of an herb employed medicinally depends on the plant. Some herbs have all or most of their medicinal substances concentrated in one part of the plant, while others have it distributed throughout. Some herbs contain more medicinal compounds in their roots, yet digging up the root destroys the plant, so the aboveground parts are used instead.

This chart of best-selling herbs gives you an idea of herb parts used.

Some Common Herbs and Their Useful Parts

Herb	Part used
Bilberry	Fruit
Echinacea	Root and/or whole flowering plant
Garlic	Clove/bulb
Ginkgo biloba	Leaves
Ginseng	Root
Goldenseal	Root
Hawthorn	Flowers, leaves, berries
Milk thistle	Seeds
Saw palmetto	Berries
St. John's wort	Flowers, whole plant

Taking charge of your health

I hope that this book will provide you the fundamental information you need to start taking charge of your own health. Notice I didn't say your own disease. If you have symptoms of a serious malady—severe pain, bleeding, neural disorders, abnormal growths, and such—then you should consult a medical doctor immediately. Conventional, or allopathic, medicine has its place, and it's the first place I'd turn if I were injured in a car wreck, for instance.

But for easing everyday problems such as headaches, insomnia, and indigestion, for keeping the body strong against potential serious diseases, and for just feeling better and more healthy and energetic on a daily basis, I know that herbs can provide wonderful benefits, and I want this book to help you learn how to take advantage of them.

If you're one of the millions of Americans who has heard that garlic can reduce your hypertension, that echinacea can make your cold go away much faster, that valerian can help you get a good night's sleep, that St. John's wort can lift your spirits, that ginkgo can improve your memory and bilberry your eyesight—but you don't know quite how to start taking advantage of these natural miracles—then I hope this book will start you on the road to better health.

Chapter 1: Dealing with the Law

One of the strongest grassroots campaigns in the history of this country resulted in the Dietary Supplement Health and Education Act (DSHEA) of 1994. The government was faced, on the one hand, with a U.S. Food and Drug Administration (FDA) initiative to control and limit consumer access to such dietary supplements as herbs and vitamins, and on the other hand, with a public outcry against such limitations. During the months that this issue was being considered, congressmen received more mail from concerned constituents than they had received on any issue in history except for the Vietnam War.

The DSHEA of 1994 allows the unrestricted sale of herbs . . . so long as medical claims are not made for these products by their manufacturer.

The resulting act bowed to the will of the people in that it allows the unrestricted sale of herbs, vitamins, minerals, and other substances such as hormones and amino acids—*so long as medical claims are not made for these products by their manufacturers.* In other words, a manufacturer may sell a product such as echinacea, which is useful against colds and flu, so long as the package doesn't say it will cure colds and flu.

Structure and function claims

So what *can* a manufacturer say about the use-fulness of a product? Descriptions of how the product affects a body's *structure* and the *function* of that structure can be made. Here are some examples.

Some Body Structures and Their Function	
Structure	**Function**
Eyes	Vision
Heart	Circulation of blood through veins and arteries
Lungs	Respiration
Prostate	Mixing of seminal fluid and sperm
Stomach and intestines	Digestion of food

According to the current DSHEA (the rules will become even more stringent next year), a product label for ginkgo can say, "Increases microcirculation to the brain." It *cannot* say, "Cures Alzheimer disease" or "Cures tinnitus". A product label for hawthorn can say, "Promotes heart health." It *cannot* say, "Cures angina pectoris."

How is the DSHEA enforced?

When any manufacturer puts a product on the market that bears a structure and/or function claim, the manufacturer must at the same time create a file of research evidence that supports the claim. The FDA has 30 days in which to investigate and challenge this evidence. Whether they choose to do so or not, the file must be available for inspection indefinitely at the manufacturer's place of business. If credible research exists, the FDA may not prohibit the manufacturer from making reasonable claims, so long as the claims are stated in terms of structure and function rather than curing disease.

> The FDA may not prohibit a manufacturer from making reasonable claims so long as they are not stated in terms of curing disease.

A recent addition to the law

Beginning in March 1998, all *new* products must not only avoid making claims about curing disease, they must not mention any disease in relation to the product—including the name. This means no tricky product names such as "ArthriCure" or "Cold-B-Gone". And after March 1999, all existing products whose name includes a disease condition must be renamed and all nutritional information must be included on the label.

Laws governing herbal supplements have become more strict, and will become even stricter in 1999.

Closing the loopholes

It's possible for a manufacturer to put out a product with structure and/or function claims that have no validity, and get by with it. It's also possible for a manufacturer to put out a useless product, make no claims for it at all, and still have unwary consumers buy it. Fortunately, the herbal- and supplement-products industries maintain self-policing organizations that informally regulate against harmful products or outright fraud.

The American Herbal Products Association (AHPA) is an association of herbalists, researchers, and manufacturers. It has created a Code of Ethics that members are expected to abide by. It also releases product safety alerts regarding adulteration of products and publishes an important reference work, the *Botanical Safety Handbook*.

> **The herbal supplement industry maintains self-policing organizations that informally regulate against harmful products or outright fraud.**

The Natural Nutritional Foods Association (NNFA) is an association of manufacturers and retailers devoted to product quality and truthful product representation. Among its many activities, the NNFA serves a strong educational role within the industry, and supports a True Label Program intended to ensure that the products put out by its members actually contain what their labels claim.

So what we have is an imperfect compromise between consumers and government regulatory agencies. Manufacturers can allude to the possible usefulness of an herb and consumers have to make personal judgements—based on research, reading, or hope—to decide which herb to use. And that's what this book is all about—helping you make the best, most informed choices possible.

CHAPTER 2: DECODING THE LABELS

I f three or four different brands or varieties of an herb are available, how do you choose which to buy? Unless you read a lot of books or magazines and get recommendations from a friend (or better yet, from a trained herbalist), you just have to do your best at deciphering the fine print on the product labels.

In thinking about how to help you understand all the intricacies of labeling practice, I went to my local health food store and selected every echinacea product available in capsule form—seven products in all. Echinacea is one of the most popular herbs, so I thought it would make a useful example. Looking at the

Of seven brands of echinacea capsules I looked at, no two were alike.

variations in content, information, terminology, manufacturing processes, claims, and dosages made me appreciate anew how confusing the world of herbal supplements has become to the consumer. Here's what I found.

- Three products were *Echinacea angustifolia*, two were *E. purpurea*, and two mixed both species. Most research has been conducted on *E. pur-*

purea, though that doesn't prove it's better.

- Two products were made from aboveground plant parts, also designated "herb" (stems, leaves, and perhaps flowers), two were made from roots and/or rhizomes, two were made from herb *and* root, and one was made from juice pressed from the flowering plant.

- Two products were standardized extracts, the other five were not. Standardized means that a product contains a certain amount of the component thought to be most medically active and that a certain percentage of the product consists of that component.

- Four products were certified organically grown, three were not.

- Six of the seven products bore batch numbers for quality control.

- Three products had "use by" dates, the others didn't.

- All the products had safety seals; two were packaged in brown glass bottles and the remainder in recyclable plastic.

- One product employed cellulose capsules for vegetarians, the remainder employed gelatin capsules.

- Capsule sizes were around 200 mg each for the standardized products, and 380 to 450 mg for whole-plant products.

- Prices for whole-plant products were $8.29, $10.49, $11.98, $15.98, and $18.95 for 100 capsules. For standardized extracts, prices were $20.95 and $21.95 for 60 capsules.

- Recommended daily dosages ranged from 1 or 2 capsules a day at the low end, to 2 to 3 capsules 2 or 3 times daily at the high end. Four products recommended discontinuing use for 2 weeks after taking the herb for 6 to 8 weeks.

- One label cautioned against use by people with autoimmune conditions, and one advised caution for pregnant women and nursing mothers.

- Some products were labeled sugar-free, one was "made with love". One was "cryogenically ground", others were harvested from the wild. In other words, these products were very inconsistent, and there was no easy way to choose among them. Reading the health claims was even more confusing. (Remember all the restrictions imposed by the DSHEA? If not, refer back to page 18.) Here's what some of the labels said (some products made no health claims at all).

- Echinacea (*Echinacea purpurea*) helps promote general well-being during the cold and flu season.*

Prices for whole-plant echinacea capsules ranged from $8.29 to $18.95 for 100 capsules

- Well researched in Europe, this herbal supplement is commonly used to promote well-being during the cold and flu season.*

- Nutritionally supports healthy immune function.*

- Echinacea is a popular herb, especially during the cold season.*

- In each case, the asterisk refers to the following statement at the bottom of the label, one that is dictated by law:

" These statements have not been evaluated by the Food and Drug Administration. This product is not intended to diagnose, treat, cure, or prevent any disease."

In fact, there's a great deal of solid research on the effectiveness of echinacea. German studies have shown that, when taken at the onset of colds or flu, it boosts the immune system by enhancing the activity of white blood cells, that during such a time it's wise to take as much as 1000 mg three times a day, and that, after taking it for two weeks, it's best to discontinue use for a few days. Too bad our current laws don't allow manufacturers to say so.

How would I choose?

Since there are so many options available, and such a lack of clear information on product packaging, here's how I would go about choosing which echinacea product to buy of those described above. Mind you, this is a personal decision, and won't necessarily be the right one for you.

First, I'd decide if I want a whole-plant product or a standardized extract. Let's say I choose whole-plant products because of the potential synergy among their various compounds. Then I'd look for a product made from the echinacea root rather than the aboveground parts, because I feel the root has higher concentrations of useful components (this is not necessarily true for other herbs). Roots are also less likely to be adulterated with other plants that look the same when dried. Products made from echinacea root tend to be more expensive, though, because the plant has to be destroyed to get it. I'd prefer a product made from *E. purpurea* to one made from *E. angustifolia*, just because most of the research has been done on the former. That doesn't mean it's better, though.

For colds or flu, it's best to take 1000 mg of echinacea three times a day— three times what some manufacturers recommend.

I'd want an organically grown product, because I'm concerned about pesticides—both for my own health and for the environment. Even though I'm a vegetarian and prefer capsules made from cellulose to ones made from animal-derived gelatin, this wouldn't determine my choice because it's too limiting.

Of the seven products I looked at, two *almost* fit my requirements. One was made from organically-grown herb *and* root of *E. purpurea*—but there's no way of knowing how much herb and how much root. One was made of the organically-grown root of *E. angustifolia*. For the same number of capsules, one cost $8.29, the other $15.98. So it would come down to weighing the value of my species of choice, amount of root, and price. What would you do?

If I had preferred a standardized extract, the choice would be less complicated. The reasons for choosing standardized might be product purity (the extracting process eliminates bacteria and fungus and other contaminants), consistency (I would know just how much of one of the major active ingredient each capsule contains), and convenience (I wouldn't need to take as many pills per day). Of the products I looked at, two were standardized to 4 percent echinacosides. Both were made from *E. angustifolia* (not my species of choice). They cost about the same ($20.95 and $21.95). I would flip a coin.

(Okay, I'll confess. What I would *really* do is choose a tincture, not a capsule, form of supplement. It would taste awful, but I feel that it would be faster-acting. That's just a personal preference.)

I wish there were some very simple rules I could give you for choosing the best herbal products. But as you can see, it's just not that simple. I can, however, give you a checklist of things to look for when you're scanning labels.

- Is the product made from the whole herb, or is it a standardized extract? (And which do you prefer?)

- Is the plant material grown organically or not? (And do you care?)

- Is the amount of active ingredient in each capsule in line with that of other similar products?

- Does the product contain any ingredients that you may be allergic to or have philosophical objections to?

- If structure and/or function health claims are made, is the appropriate disclaimer regarding the FDA included?

- Is the package safely sealed?

- Is there an expiration date on the product, and is it in the future?

- Is there a batch number on the product in case you want to ask the manufacturer about it?

- Does the manufacturer list an address, telephone number, or website address so you can get more information?

- Is the price consistent with that of other similar products, or if it's more expensive, is there an obvious reason?

When you're selecting herbal products, my best advice is to take a magnifying glass along! Those labels are hard to read!

A Typical Label
Front

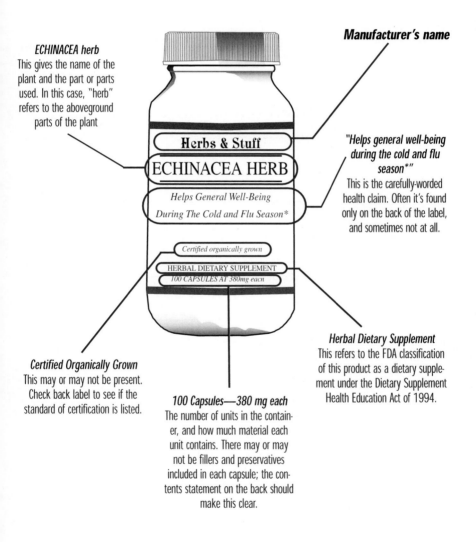

ECHINACEA herb
This gives the name of the plant and the part or parts used. In this case, "herb" refers to the aboveground parts of the plant

Manufacturer's name

Herbs & Stuff

ECHINACEA HERB

*Helps General Well-Being During The Cold and Flu Season**

Certified organically grown

HERBAL DIETARY SUPPLEMENT

100 CAPSULES AT 380mg each

"Helps general well-being during the cold and flu season*"
This is the carefully-worded health claim. Often it's found only on the back of the label, and sometimes not at all.

Certified Organically Grown
This may or may not be present. Check back label to see if the standard of certification is listed.

100 Capsules—380 mg each
The number of units in the container, and how much material each unit contains. There may or may not be fillers and preservatives included in each capsule; the contents statement on the back should make this clear.

Herbal Dietary Supplement
This refers to the FDA classification of this product as a dietary supplement under the Dietary Supplement Health Education Act of 1994.

A Typical Label
Side

*Echinacea (Echinacea purpurea) helps promote general well-being during the cold and flu season.** The health claim. After March 1998 this statement will not be allowed—even if it has been proven true— because it refers to disease.

Our Echinacea purpurea is Organically Grown by Smith Farms and Certified Organically Processed in accordance with Oregon Tilth standards and the California Organic Foods Act of 1990. Most organic products that are certified are processed in accordance with the standards spelled out in the California Organic Foods Act of 1990. Organic growing standards vary from one part of the country to another, but uniform laws are under discussion.

> **Echinacea** (*Echinacea purperea*) helps promote general well-being during the cold and flu season*
>
> Echinacea grows wild in the midwest, and was used by Native Americans more than any other herb. Today echinacea is the best known herb available. It has received positive reviews from doctors on national television. In Germany, it is one of the most researched herbs available. Its benefits have been shown in many European clinical studies
>
> *Our Echinacea purpurea is Organically Grown by Smith Farms and Certified Organically Processed in accordance with Oregon Tilth standards and the California Organic Foods Act of 1990.*
>
> * These statements have not been evaluated by the Food and Drug Administration. This product is not intended to diagnose, treat, cure, or prevent any disease.
>
> Manufactured by Herbs & Stuff, PO Box 0000, Somewhere, USA, 80001
>
> 1997 R/1

Echinacea grows wild in the midwest, and was used by Native Americans more than any other herb. Today echinacea is the best known herb available. It has received positive reviews from doctors on national television. In Germany, it is one of the most researched herbs available. Its benefits have been shown in many European clinical studies. This kind of background information may or may not be included on a product. It is interesting and helps build credibility.

Manufacturer Address Inclusion of an address is required by law. It's also a convenience to the consumer in contacting the manufacturer with questions or complaints. This part of the label might also read "Distributed by", in which case you might be left wondering who actually made the product.

1997 R/1 This shows that the text on the label has been copyrighted by the manufacturer.

***These statements have not been evaluated by the Food and Drug Administration. This product is not intended to diagnose, treat, cure, or prevent any disease.* This statement is required on any product that makes a structure and function or health claim. However, it's a fairly recent requirement, and products that don't carry it may predate the law.

A Typical Label
Other Side and Bottom

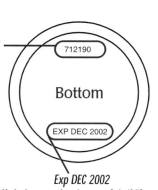

Recommendation: As an addition to the daily diet, take one to three capsules three times daily, preferably with food. After taking Echinacea for 6 to 8 weeks, a two-week break is recommended before restarting use for best results.

The manufacturer's recommended dosages vary from one product to another, particularly on non-standardized products. It's generally a good practice to follow them—though in the case of echinacea, much more can and probably should be taken when a cold is coming on.

Recommendation: As an addition to the daily diet, take one to three capsules three times daily, preferably with food. After taking Echinacea for 6 to 8 weeks, a two-week break is recommended before restarting use for best results.

Caution: Not recommended for individuals with auto-immune conditions.

Double safety-sealed with a printed outer shrinkwrap film and a printed inner bottle freshness seal. Do not use if either seal is broken or missing.

Caution: Not recommended for individuals with auto-immune conditions.

It's always wise to observe manufacturer's cautions. In the case of echinacea, which is known as an immune stimulant, the message here is that it hasn't been shown to help such conditions as lupus and AIDS. Furthermore, it may be harmful for a condition such as chronic fatigue syndrome, in which the immune system's balance is precarious.

Double safety-sealed with a printed outer shrinkwrap film and a printed inner bottle freshness seal. Do not use if either seal is broken or missing.

This is the same kind of caution that appears on all over-the-counter medications, and many foods, today.

712190

The batch number. Manufacturers keep a portion of each batch in inventory, so that if any problems are reported, they can go back and analyze it.

712190

Bottom

EXP DEC 2002

Exp DEC 2002

This speaks for itself. Herbs have varying degrees of shelf life, and ones that are sealed and kept away from light and heat tend to retain their benefits for quite a while.

Chapter 3: Deciding Which Supplement Form to Use

Not only are hundreds of different herbs available in the marketplace, they come in a bewildering variety of forms. Should you buy a tea, a tincture, a capsule? Which is better, or does it matter? Understanding the different preparations and how they're made will help you make informed choices.

> ## Should you buy a tea, a tincture, a capsule? Which is better, or does it matter?

If I seem to be emphasizing capsules in this discussion, it's because that's the form in which 80 percent of all herbal supplements are sold. This is not because they are necessarily better. They are, however, convenient and palatable.

Echinacea—a case study

Let's look at a single familiar herb, echinacea. It can be prepared in any of the following ways, and these do not exhaust all the possibilities.

- Harvest and dry all aboveground parts (stems, leaves, flowers), grind and sift, and form into tablets or capsules.

- Harvest and dry the roots, grind and sift, and form into tablets or capsules.

- Harvest flowering plants and press the juices from them while they're fresh. This form of echinacea was used in a positive test conducted by the German Commission E, a regulatory agency responsible for approving herbal medicines in that country.

- Grind, crush, and mill the root, soak it in alcohol to dissolve out some or all of the active ingredients, strain, and use the liquid. (Water or glycerine may be substituted for alcohol, but the resulting product may not have the same kind or amount of active ingredients.)

- Grind, crush, and mill the root or whole plant, treat with a solvent such as acetone or ketone, which will bind with some of the chemical compounds in the plant material. Wash out the unbonded solvent and form the remaining substance into capsules or tablets.

All these processes result in products with some active ingredients that can stimulate the immune system against colds and flu. But which is better? Is there really any way to know? One of the biggest controversies among herbalists and medicinal manufacturers is whether preparations made from whole herbs are superior to extracts, and whether whole-herb extracts are superior to standardized ones. The examples above are a continuum. The first two provide a product that contains the whole plant or a major portion of it. The third provides the juice of the whole plant. The fourth provides those chemical compounds in the plant that are soluble in alcohol. The last is the least natural, the most laboratory-controlled. By selective use of various solvents, the manufacturer controls which plant compounds are extracted—in the case of echinacea, echinosides—and how many of them end up in the final product.

> **One of the biggest controversies among herbalists and medicinal manufacturers is whether preparations made from whole herbs are superior to extracts, and whether whole-herb extracts are superior to standardized ones**

Those who advocate whole-herb preparations argue that there are many, many compounds in any given herb, and that they act synergistically to provide the maximum benefit to the user. Those who advocate standardized extracts argue that without a rigorous process of concentrating and measuring one or more compounds in the product, you don't really know what you're getting.

Both are right.

Whole herb vs. extract?

The concentration of medicinal compounds in herbs varies a lot from one kind of plant to another. For instance, a teaspoon of dried pepper- mint leaves is powerful enough to make a tea

Are standardized products superior to unstandardized ones? Not necessarily.

that's very effective in calming an upset stomach. But a tea made from a teaspoon of ginkgo leaves would have no value at all in restoring your memo- ry. It takes many, many pounds of ginkgo leaves to make a single effective dose (and the doses must be repeated regularly over time).

So how do you know if the ginkgo product you've just bought is concentrated enough to do any good? The manufacturer probably has standardized it. For ginkgo, standardization means that a product contains approximately 24% glycosides.

Most herbs that are standardized don't require the extreme concentration that ginkgo does, and, in fact, are often standardized for other reasons. Perhaps a single component has been isolated for research, and the manufacturer wants to be sure that the amount on which research was conducted is found in the product. Does this make that product superior to others which are not standardized? Not necessarily. But standardizing does give some assurance of content and benefit.

The chart on page 41 shows other often-used herbs that are usually standardized, the component that is identified for standardization, and the amount of that component you'll find in most products.

Other forms of herbs

Spray. This relatively new form of supplement is a liquid which is sprayed under the tongue. The active ingredients enter the blood stream quickly,

Some Commonly Standardized Herbs

Most herbalists will recommend that you take herbs as whole herbs, not standardized forms. But most herbal medicines have been investigated as standardized supplements. Here are some of the herbs I favor in standardized form, and the percentages of particular compounds they usually contain.

Bilberry	25% anthocyanocides
Garlic	5.4 mg allicin dose
Ginkgo biloba	24% ginkgo flavone glycosides, 6% terpene lactones
Grapeseed	95% proanthocyanidins
Hawthorn	3.2% vitexin
Kava-kava	29% kavalactones
Licorice	2% glycyrrhizin
Milk thistle	70% silymarin
Saw palmetto	95% free fatty acids
St John's wort	.3–.5% hypericin

bypassing the gastrointestinal tract where they might be damaged by stomach acids. This form is useful for people who have difficulty swallowing tablets or capsules.

Tablet. A carefully controlled quantity of finely milled herbal material is compressed into the chosen shape and given a thin coating. Enteric coatings are formulated in such a way that they do not dissolve until the tablet reaches the small intestine, where it can be absorbed without being affected by stomach acids. Some tablets are made to dissolve under the tongue, where absorption into the bloodstream is rapid.

Tea. This is the most familiar, most traditional herbal preparation. What you buy is dried plant material—leaf, flower, bark, root, seed, berry. What you do with it is use hot water to extract some of the material's active components. Some herbs lend themselves very well to this process. Peppermint, chamomile, and sage are examples of herbs that release their volatile oils readily in near-boiling water. Others—ginkgo leaf, for example—could be boiled all day and not yield anything useful. Hard or woody plant parts need longer steeping or soaking to make an effective tea.

Tincture. The active compounds in some herbs are not water soluble, so they are steeped in alcohol instead, the result being a simple extract. Tinctures are sometimes called extracts or liquid extracts. They are generally taken in small amounts—droppersful or teaspoonsful—mixed with water.

Chapter 4: How Supplements are Manufactured

We've come to depend on the federal government to approve and police the contents and safety of the medicines we use, whether we get them by prescription or over the counter. But by classifying herbal medicines as dietary supplements instead of medicines, the Dietary Supplement Health Education Act of 1994 (DSHEA) has shifted a lot of responsibility for product quality to the manufacturers.

Does that make you nervous? Mistakes do happen, and not everyone adheres to the same standards. Fortunately, a lot of safeguards help ensure product integrity.

In the first place, the Food and Drug Administration (FDA) does regulate the way that herbal products are manufactured. They have a checklist of good manufacturing procedures that must be strictly adhered to. And some herbal-product manufacturers have decided to adopt even stricter manufacturing procedures—more like those used in the pharmaceutical industry.

Second, the herbal-supplement industry has some self-policing programs such as the True Labels program of the National Natural Foods Association and the watchdog activities of the

American Herbal Products Association (see page 115). These voluntary initiatives are intended to help ensure that the products you buy will be what's represented on their labels.

Finally, most manufacturers use rigorous testing programs from start to finish. I've visited several supplement manufacturers and have been impressed and reassured by what I've seen. Here's a typical life history of a typical herb capsule.

Most major manufacturers observe food or pharmaceutical standards in their manufacturing process.

Identification and testing. When herbal material arrives at the factory in sacks or bales or drums, samples are taken to the laboratory for identification. The first identification process is organoleptic—a fancy name for smelling it, tasting it, and looking at it under the microscope. In most labs, the sample also is subjected to high-performance liquid chromatography. This sophisticated test identifies the herb and indicates its quality by profiling its chemical compounds.

Quarantine. While the sample is being tested, the bulk of the material is quarantined. Raw materials from outside the country may be quarantined for as long as six months; for domestic herbs, the quarantine is usually shorter. Once quarantine is over, the herb is tested again, cleaned, and made ready for processing. In some cases the material is heat-treated to kill bacteria and other microorganisms.

> **Raw herbs from outside the country may be quarantined for as long as six months before being processed.**

Milling. After testing, quarantine, and cleaning, the herbal material is milled (ground) into a fine powder. This is done in such a way that its temperature isn't raised too high, because heat can destroy important plant compounds. Once the herb has been milled to a fine powder, it may be stored for future use or made into capsules, pills, or tinctures. (Many manufacturers buy their herbs in milled form from large product wholesalers, who will have done their own testing and passed the results on to the manufacturer.)

Encapsulation. Capsules can be made by hand with very simple equipment, but larger manufacturers use sophisticated encapsulating machines that can produce thousands of capsules an hour. These semi-automatic machines are housed in rooms whose temperature, pressure, dust, and humidity can be controlled. The only human interaction with the machine is watching raw material loaded into the hoppers.

Inspection. After the capsules are made, they ride a conveyer belt for visual inspection. Any faulty capsules—ones that are cracked, broken, or not completely filled—are discarded.

Packaging. Capsules that pass inspection are fed into bottles by machines that count their number, safety-seal the bottles, stamp on batch numbers and expiration dates, and attach labels. A quality check completes the packaging process.

Keeping records. In case there are reports of problems, manufacturers keep and store a sample from each batch of herbal preparation. This is important insurance for the consumer. In the

unlikely case of product adulteration, the manufacturer will be able to test the stored sample to
analyze the problem and will know which batch or
batches to recall.

A full year or more can elapse from the time
herbal material is harvested until the finished product finds its way to the shelf of your health-food
store. It's a long and demanding process, with testing occurring at every stage. Because the raw
materials of herb supplements are so variable,
ensuring a consistent finished product is much
more difficult than it is with chemical drugs that are
synthesized in a laboratory. Understanding this
process should help you ask the kind of questions
of your local retailer or the manufacturer that will
give you confidence in your products of choice.

A SELECTED LIST OF MANUFACTURERS

I'm sure there are others who are equally good, but I can personally recommend products from the following manufacturers. I've tried their products and visited many of their facilities. They all observe Good Manufacturing Processes (GMP), and many go even further by adhering to Food or Pharmaceutical manufacturing standards. Call their customer service hot-lines or visit their websites for more information, or look for their products at your favorite herb retail store.

Action Labs	800-932-2953	
Alvita Teas	800-258-4828	www.naturesherbs.com
Celestial Seasonings	800-498-8004	www.celestialseasonings.com
Enzymatic Therapy	800-783-2286	www.enzy.com
Flora	800-446-2110	www.florainc.com
Frontier Herbs	800-669-3275	www.frontiercoop.com
Futurebiotics	800-367-5433	www.futurebiotics.com
Gaia Herbs	800-831-7780	
Herb Pharm	800-348-4372	
Herbs Etc.	800-634-3727	
Herbal Plus	888-462-2548	www.gnc.com
KAL	800-579-4665	
Natrol	800-326-1520	www.natrol.com
Nature's Fingerprint	888-462-2548	www.gnc.com
Nature's Herbs	800-437-2257	www.naturesherbs.com
Nature's Plus	800-645-9500	www.natplus.com
Nature's Resource	800-314-4372	
Nature's Way	800-962-8873	www.naturesway.com
Rainbow Light	800-635-1233	
Schiff	800-526-6251	www.weider.com
Solaray	800-579-4665	
Solgar	800-645-2246	www.solgar.com

CHAPTER 5: CAUTIONS ABOUT USING HERBS

Most common medicinal herbs, and especially those that have been converted into well-tested supplements, are relatively safe for most people when taken as directed. At the same time, it's important for you to learn as much as you can about all the supplements that you plan on taking and to use a lot of common sense to avoid possible allergic reactions, or harmful interactions with existing conditions or medications. I advise, when trying a new herbal supplement, that you start out with the recommended dose and monitor your responses very closely.

> When trying a new herbal supplement, start out with the recommended dose and monitor your responses closely.

Allergies

Some people have allergic reactions to plant foods or airborne plant substances. Since herbs are both plants and food, and herbal supplements may be very concentrated, it's not unheard of for allergic reactions to occur. There are some common-sense predictors. If you're allergic to ragweed, you will want to be cautious about using chamomile, which is also in the aster plant family. Monitor yourself when trying a new herbal supplement, and if you have any unpleasant side effects such as rashes, dizziness, nausea, or headaches, stop taking the supplement immediately.

Food and drug interactions

We also know that some herbs can interact in negative ways with certain foods, pharmaceutical drugs, caffeine, or alcohol. Read your labels. If you're using any of these substances, be careful about adding a herb that could cause a critical interaction.

Common sense is useful here, too. If you have high blood pressure, don't take an herb such as ephedra that elevates the blood pressure. If you have thin blood that doesn't clot readily, don't take an herb such as garlic that thins the blood. If you are a bundle of nerves from drinking too much coffee, don't take an herb such as green tea that is loaded with caffeine. The longest list of "don'ts" probably applies to pregnant and nursing women. Many common herbs are smooth-muscle relaxants, and can interfere with the tone of uterine muscles and even lead to premature delivery. Other herbs can cross the placenta and give the fetus a dose of something it doesn't need! Likewise, many herbs show up in a mother's milk. I've heard of babies getting garlic breath when they nurse! This isn't necessarily a bad thing, but some herbs can be harmful to babies. Check the list on page 83 if you're pregnant or nursing.

Observing dosage recommendations

Virtually every report in recent years about harmful effects of herbs has stemmed from cases in which people didn't follow directions. A young person died from an overdose of ephedra a couple of years ago, but he had consumed an extraordinary quantity, far beyond label recommendations. Another person was arrested for erratic driving after taking a large amount of kava-kava. Again, he had far exceeded label recommendations. An elderly woman died from pennyroyal poisoning a number of years ago, but she had taken a great deal of straight essential oil—something no label, book, or herbal practitioner would ever recommend. Dosage recommendations on reliable products are safe and even conservative. Don't second-guess them unless you have good advice from a trained herbalist.

Following manufacturers' instructions is important. If a tincture says, "take 30 drops in water", don't just squirt it in your mouth straight. I have a colleague who did that with echinacea during a bad cold. The alcohol in the extract irritated the inflamed tissues of her throat, causing it to swell shut. This was an unusual reaction, but it's best to be on the safe side. Furthermore, those extracts can taste pretty disagreeable by themselves. You might want to try juice instead of water.

Supplement manufacturers tend to be very careful and conservative in making dosage recommendations, and it's wise to follow label instructions. One thing the labels won't tell you, though, is that most supplements are formulated for the needs of a 150-pound man. If you're much heavier or lighter than that, consider adjusting your dose accordingly.

Know your sources

Make sure that you're buying herbal supplements from a quality manufacturer or other herbal provider whom you can trust. I feel comfortable recommending the major manufacturers of herbal products in this country. I have visited many of their factories and can vouch for their high standards and attention to quality. I would be wary of products that are unusually inexpensive or promoted by companies that make excessive claims. It's also good to shop for herbal products in retail stores that stand behind the products. Most retailers do a good job of researching the manufacturers whose products they sell.

I've attended the major trade shows that represent all the reputable manufacturers of herbal products in America and I've found a high degree of concern about product quality. Nowadays more and more mass merchandisers are jumping into the sale of herbal supplements. It's important to make sure that you compare and closely read the labels on all these products. There are good and bad buys available everywhere. Use the information in this book to read labels knowledgeably. Become a good herbal shopper.

Seek expert advice

I always tell people receiving other medical therapy to check with their health-care provider when they start taking any herbal supplements. The biggest problem with this advice is that most medical doctors have limited knowledge of herbal supplements and their interactions with prescription medicines. Fortunately, trained herbalists are becoming more numerous, and some conventional health-care providers are learning about the benefits of herbal supplements. But because herbal medication is often self-medication, it's important that you know enough to treat yourself the way you wish a doctor would. With authority, insight, and precision.

Dangerous herbs

The following herbs should be avoided altogether or used only under the supervision of a health-care professional.

American mistletoe
Belladonna
Chaparral
Comfrey
Foxglove
Madagascar periwinkle
Mandrake
Mayapple
Pennyroyal
Pokeweed
Rue
Tansy
Yohimbe

CHAPTER 6: **GETTING STARTED**

To feel well, age gracefully, correct minor health problems—these are some of the best reasons to use herbs in your day-to-day life. You can learn enough about herbs on your own to make a real difference. However, using herbs for serious health problems instead of going to a qualified health practitioner—whether a trained herbalist or a medical doctor—is not what I'll be advocating in this part of the book.

Here I want to help you get started with herbal wellness in a conservative, responsible way by describing some of the health problems that can be avoided or improved with herbal supplements. I'll say right here that I don't have formal training in either herbalism or conventional medicine (except for an advanced degree in clinical psychology). I have, however, spent a lot of time and effort over the last dozen years researching, reading, and trying herbs on my own. The information I'll be presenting is backed by current research and the best information I have gleaned from professionals in the herb industry, tempered with my own experience.

In fact, I'd like to start with this experience as an example of how an ordinary person can use herbal supplements for better health. At age 49 I have no serious health problems. I eat healthy foods, exercise regularly, and don't smoke. In fact, I'm very healthy—but I haven't always been. Twelve years ago I had high blood pressure, high cholesterol, stomach and digestive problems, and low energy. I decided to change my lifestyle and eating habits, and for the last three years I've also been taking tonic herbs.

My wellness routine includes ginkgo biloba for memory and vision, saw palmetto for my prostate, garlic to keep my blood pressure and cholesterol low, Siberian ginseng for energy and overall well-being, bilberry for eyesight and circulation, milk thistle for my liver, and kelp to stimulate my thyroid. (In addition to these herbs, I also take an iron-free multivitamin, Coenzyme Q10 for my heart, and extra vitamins C and E and selenium as antioxidants.) I know this sounds like a lot, but my health is very important to me and I've come to believe in the value of these supplements in maintaining health. I'm seldom ill and have loads of energy.

In addition to these "insurance" supplements, I also take herbs to prevent or cure minor illnesses when I feel I'm getting sick. During the cold and flu season, if I get a sniffle or a tingle of a sore throat,

I start immediately with elderberry and echinacea in large doses throughout the day. This regimen has definitely helped me, sometimes stopping a cold dead before it starts.

I've learned what's right for me through trial and error. It's up to you to decide how far you want to go with treating your problems with herbal medicine and how responsible you want to be for your own health.

Don't Take Chances

I can't emphasize enough how important it is to check with a qualified health-care provider before you decide to treat any serious illness on your own or to take any herbs that could interact negatively with drugs prescribed for you. I make this recommendation with the full knowledge that your health-care provider may know nothing about herbal supplements and may be totally against their use. You can help educate your health-care provider by furnishing him or her with good solid information about the health benefits of herbal supplements, using some of the reference materials listed at the end of this book. You may also wish to consult these references yourself.

Conditions Requiring Immediate Medical Attention

This book helps you choose the best herbal products, but it is not in any way meant to replace doctors or the medical profession. If you have any of the following symptoms or problems, see your health-care provider immediately.

Allergic reaction
Back injury
Bleeding that won't stop
Blood in the stool
Blood in the urine
Chest pains
Dizziness or disorientation
Drowsiness, stupor, or unconsciousness
Head injury
Heart palpitations or irregular heartbeat
High blood pressure
High fever
Poisoning
Serious infection
Severe pains
Shortness of breath
Sudden loss of physical functioning
Unusual lumps or growths

Chapter 7: Using Tonic Herbs and Antioxidants

As a society, we're beginning to focus on wellness more than on illness. This change is partly a result of the health-care industry and the emergence of managed-care organizations. But more important, it's because we're an aging population that wants to live well in our later years. More of us are focusing on diet, exercise, and general fitness. Using herbs to build and sustain good health is as logical as it is smart.

It's generally accepted that most peoples' diets don't supply all the nutrients necessary for optimum health. (How many of us really eat five servings of vegetables and seven servings of grains every single day?) If you take vitamins to supplement your imperfect diet, it's probably not because you're afraid of getting scurvy or rickets. It's because you want to sustain a high level of health and well-being. I feel that taking certain herbs routinely is just as important as taking vitamins A, B, and C.

We're an aging population that wants to live well in our later years.

The herbs that I incorporate into my daily routine, every day of the year, are from the classes of tonic herbs and antioxidants. These can be beneficial to anybody regardless of age or condition; you can take them forever with no bad side effects. I think of them as a nutritional insurance policy.

Ginseng has a long history of use, but no one has been able to prove precisely what it does.

Tonic herbs

Look up "tonic" in the dictionary, and you'll see synonyms such as restorative, invigorant, stimulant, booster, refresher. The best known tonic herb in the Western world is probably ginseng. It's also been one of the most controversial, because it has a long history of use, but no one has been able to prove precisely what it does. That's because its action is *nonspecific*. It doesn't cure any particular disease in any measurable way. But it does enhance energy and general health, improve concentration and sensory discrimination, and subtly regulate a range of body functions—metabolism, blood pressure, oxygen uptake, and more. It sounds miraculous, doesn't it?

And there are other herbs that have the same benefits—Siberian ginseng (eleuthero), mushrooms such as maitake and reishi, and gotu kola, to name a few. You might see these also referred to as *adaptogens*, which means that they build resistance to physical stress by strengthening the immune, nervous, and/or glandular systems. Sure, you can be a healthy, vigorous individual without taking them, but why not optimize your odds?

> Adaptogens are herbs that build resistance to physical stress by strengthening the immune, nervous, and/or glandular systems.

Antioxidants

It's natural for our bodies to age. Normal metabolism causes the creation of free radicals, which in turn cause general aging, cell degeneration, and disease. At the same time, it's natural for our bodies to produce antioxidants that neutralize these free radicals—*if* we give our bodies the right nutrients to work with. And that's the catch. Antioxidants are present in fresh fruits and vegetables and in other whole foods, but the average American diet doesn't offer enough of them. So supplementation is important.

Antioxidants neutralize free radicals which cause aging, cell degeneration, and disease.

Vitamins C and E have strong antioxidant properties, as do such minerals as selenium—but certain herbs are even better. Green tea, grapeseed extract, and rosemary are all extraordinarily effective antioxidants and provide great insurance against many of the degenerative conditions that we all want to postpone or avoid.

Other preventives

There are other herbs that have good, general preventive effects that don't fit neatly into either of the categories above. Some can be classified as tonics or adaptogens, some have antioxidant properties, but they also have more specific effects on certain body systems, either as preventives or curatives. These include the herbs that I take every

Herbs for General Wellness

American ginseng	General tonic, adaptogen
Astragalus	General tonic; boosts energy
Bilberry	Improves circulation, repairs veins
Chinese ginseng	General tonic; boosts energy
Garlic	Lowers cholesterol; anticancer agent
Grapeseed extract	Antioxidant
Ginkgo biloba	Antioxidant; improves circulation and memory
Gotu kola	Improves circulation, healing, memory
Green tea	Antioxidant, anticancer agent, tonic
Maitake	Tonic, anticancer agent; enhances immune system
Milk thistle	Liver tonic
Reishi	Adaptogen, tonic, immunostimulant
Siberian ginseng	Adaptogen, tonic; boosts energy
Turmeric	Antioxidant

day—ginkgo biloba for brain function, bilberry for eyesight, milk thistle for the liver, garlic for high blood pressure and high cholesterol. You'll read more about them in later chapters, but they fit well here as preventives, too.

Chapter 8: USING HERBS TO STAY WELL

Coughs, sniffles, aches and pains are part of life. They usually signal problems that are bothersome but not life-threatening. If you go to your doctor with problems such as a common cold, minor arthritic pain (what used to be called "rheumatism"), or restless nights, you're likely to get little or no help—or else more help than you want (and need) with pharmaceutical drugs and their unpleasant side effects.

Some of these minor problems are a predictable part of growing old. While anybody can experience an upset stomach or heartburn, constipation is more likely to become a frequent problem in later years. That's true for sleep disorders as well. And while ear infections are common among infants and toddlers whose Eustachian tubes are immature, tinnitus is most often a problem—and a very annoying one—among the elderly.

Treating these annoying but not life-threatening problems with medicinal herbs is often more helpful than a trip to your doctor.

Colds and flu

No other health problem results in as much lost work time or as many dollars spent at pharmacies the common cold and flu. Yet there's little that a medical doctor can do to treat these conditions but suggest aspirin and prescribe an antibiotic (which usually doesn't help, since most colds and flu are viral in origin). The world of herbal medicine has a better answer, and there's good research to prove its effectiveness: echinacea.

Many clinical studies in Europe have shown that taking large doses of echinacea at the onset of cold and flu symptoms will reduce the duration of the illness from ten days to four. I can say from personal experience and that of many acquaintances that if you start early enough, you can avoid the cold or flu altogether. That's because echinacea stimulates the activity of disease-fighting cells in the blood.

Treating annoying but not life-threatening problems with medicinal herbs is often more helpful than a trip to your doctor.

You'll often find echinacea combined with goldenseal in herbal products. There has been less research done on goldenseal, but it is known to

soothe inflammation of the mucous membranes—
a great boon for cold sufferers.

Garlic, in addition to all its other useful properties, is a powerful antibacterial agent. Ask experienced herbalists what they do at the onset of a
cold, and nine times out of ten you'll hear "start
taking large amounts of
garlic." That can mean
whole garlic capsules if
you're concerned about
offensive breath, or raw
garlic cloves if you're not.
Garlic, echinacea, and
goldenseal are a power-
ful trio during cold and
flu season.

No matter which
herbal cold remedy
you select, it's
important to take
enough at the
right time.

A fourth member of
the cold and flu arsenal is
elderberry (*Sambucus nigra*). There is a relatively
new herbal product on the market, primarily made
of the juice of the elderberry, for which exciting
research has been conducted in Israel during the
past three or four years. What elderberry seems to
do is prevent cold- and flu-causing microorganisms
from taking hold in throat tissues. Maybe like me,

you've experienced the cold that starts in your sinuses and moves down into your throat, and maybe from there to your chest and back up. Elderberry products show great promise in preventing this miserable journey.

No matter which herbal cold remedy you select, it's important to take enough at the right time. I know lots of people who, when they feel a cold coming on, take a couple of echinacea tablets. Guess what—that doesn't do any good! Herbs aren't like aspirin. You need lots to make an effect. Check the dosage recommendations in the table at the end of this chapter.

Finally, if you haven't been able to avoid that miserable cold, and you're fighting sinusitis, nasal congestion, and headache, consider ephedra (called ma huang in Traditional Chinese Medicine). Taken according to manufacturers' recommendations, ephedra is a gentle, effective decongestant with fewer unpleasant side effects than over-the-counter pharmaceutical preparations. It's gotten some bad press in recent years because it can be abused (kids have taken it to get high; in one case, a teenager died). But used responsibly, ephedra is a fine addition to the herbal arsenal for colds and flu. It should not be used by anyone with high blood pressure or anyone taking prescription medications.

For your digestive tract

Heartburn. Gas. Queasiness. Almost everyone has these problems from time to time, and for some people they're chronic. A number of gentle, effective herbal remedies are worth trying. Leading the list for general digestive problems, in my experience, is peppermint. A simple cup of peppermint tea after a meal is amazingly calming. Aloe calms an inflamed stomach. And for motion sickness (or other situations that produce nausea), ginger is an excellent alternative to chemical treatments.

As we age, the smooth muscles of the small and large intestines tend to get lazy. The result is often constipation. This can be more than annoying—sluggish bowels lead to other more serious conditions such as diverticulitis. Nature provides some excellent plant remedies: cascara sagrada, the husks of psyllium seed, and flaxseed. We don't always think of these last two as herbs, but they fit my definition—plants with specific medicinal benefits.

Stressed? Can't sleep?

It's the rare adult in this day and age who doesn't suffer from stress and stress-related conditions. I'll talk about serious problems such as high blood pressure and ulcers in the next chapter, but here I'd like to say a word in favor of treating the cause. Not so long ago, it was common for people to take prescribed tranquilizers and "downers" to offset the stresses in their lives. We've learned a lot in recent years about the dangers of this practice, in terms of addiction and impaired quality of life. Fortunately, there are herbal alternatives with few or no side effects, among them the time-honored calmatives chamomile, kava-kava, and valerian.

Sleepless nights can be a problem at any age, especially if you lead a demanding life. But as we grow older, interrupted sleep often becomes more of a problem. Valerian is among the most effective herbs for promoting good sleep; you can also take passionflower or a simple cup of chamomile tea. Valerian has the interesting property of being extremely bad-smelling. I've even heard people say they bought some, thought it was spoiled, and threw it away. My advice is hold your nose and swallow for a good night's sleep.

Herbs for Minor Conditions

For colds and flu	
Astragalus	1000 mg 3 times a day before symptoms become acute
Echinacea	1000 mg 3 times a day
Elderberry	3 tablespoons syrup a day
Garlic	900 mg of .6% allicin a day
Goldenseal	1000 mg 3 times a day when fever is present
For digestion	
Ginger	3000 mg 3 times a day
Peppermint	1000 mg as a tea 3 times a day
For constipation	
Cascara sagrada	1 ml with 1 cup water daily
Psyllium	1 teaspoon with 1 cup water daily

For anxiety and stress	
Hops	1 teaspoon in a cup of water as tea daily as needed
Kava-kava	1000 mg 3 times a day
Passionflower	1 teaspoon in a cup of water as tea daily as needed
Valerian	300–400 mg daily as needed

For insomnia	
Chamomile	1 teaspoon in a cup of water as tea before bed
Hops	1 teaspoon in a cup of water as tea before bed
Valerian	300–400 mg before bed

CHAPTER 9: USING HERBS TO AVOID SERIOUS PROBLEMS

In the last chapter we talked about some fairly common, aggravating, but non-life-threatening conditions for which herbs can provide help. Here we're walking a narrower line. There are serious medical conditions such as hypertension, high cholesterol, and benign prostatic hyperplasia for which solidly researched and effective herbal treatments, especially preventive ones, do exist. There are other conditions, such as diabetes and Alzheimer disease, for which certain herbs may be useful by themselves or in conjunction with conventional medical treatment, but for which research has not been conclusive.

The fact is, there's an herbal remedy of some sort for just about every medical problem that exists. After all, herbs are all that our ancestors had to work with and they found that some herbs were

> There are serious medical conditions such as hypertension, high cholesterol, and benign prostatic hyperplasia for which solidly researched and effective herbal treatments, especially preventive ones, do exist.

more effective than others. With today's herbal choices, you need to decide what your personal comfort zone is and seek information that will help you make good choices.

For myself, I like to consider the amount of risk involved in both the disease and the treatment. What's the very worst that can happen? On one end of the continuum, maybe it's nothing. On the other end, maybe it's death. In between, effects may range from a simple upset stomach to a serious loss of function. If the risk to trying an herbal treatment falls within my comfort zone, then I want to know the documented evidence for the treatment's success. Is there solid scientific evidence? Or is it all testimonials and hearsay? Is the documented success rate one out of a hundred, or one out of two?

The most threatening diseases—cancer, stroke, dementia, Parkinson disease—are far beyond the scope of this book. But there are many conditions that can seriously affect your quality of life for which herbs can provide relief or prevention.

Healthy eyes and ears
Diminished eyesight is an almost inevitable part of aging, even for those of us who have had

good vision throughout our early lives. Bilberry is a simple herbal assistant for vision problems that stem from poor circulation to the eyes. While it has been studied particularly for its vision benefits, bilberry also increases circulation in other parts of the body, making it useful in helping or preventing minor varicose veins. You have to take it indefinitely, though—if you quit, the benefits quit, too.

The nutrients in bilberry increase the retinin that enables you to see, particularly at night, while ginkgo helps prevent macular degeneration by increasing blood flow to the eye. European researchers have studied the effects of both herbs on vision and report promising results when they're taken together.

Tinnitus (ringing in the ears) may not sound serious—unless you suffer from it. If you do, ginkgo biloba can bring relief. And since ginkgo is important for brain function (see below), and has no negative side effects, taking it is good overall insurance.

Healthy internal organs

There's been a history of heart disease in my family, so even though my heart is perfectly healthy, I take hawthorn every day. It has a long history in western European herbalism as a heart strengthener, and some studies have shown that it can help relieve angina pectoris and prevent congestive heart failure. If you suffer from heart disease, you *must* seek expert medical care. But if heart problems are something you're trying to avoid, as I am, a daily dose of hawthorn is a smart preventive.

We hear less about diseases of the liver than of the heart, but they are no less serious. The irreplaceable liver is essential for digestion and cleaning toxins from the blood. If you're suffering from any form of liver disease, you *must* seek expert medical advice. If you're not, a regular dose of milk thistle will stimulate the liver and keep it doing its job efficiently. With all the pollutants our bodies have to deal with (including the ones we inflict on ourselves, such as alcohol), and the threat of serious chronic liver diseases such as hepatitis C

With all the pollutants our bodies have to deal with, it makes good sense to use every preventive measure possible.

and cirrhosis, it makes good sense to use every preventive measure possible—including milk thistle, which is widely prescribed in Europe for liver problems.

A healthy brain—and mind

One of the greatest fears associated with aging is loss of mental function. And as people in our society live longer and longer, conditions such as Alzheimer disease become more and more of a threat. It's a little-understood disease with devastating effects on both victims and their families—so you're well advised to practice prevention.

> Ginkgo biloba is one of the leading herbal prescriptions in Europe, and it's becoming one of the best-selling herbal supplements in the United States.

Ginkgo biloba is one of the leading herbal prescriptions in Europe, and it's becoming one of the best-selling herbal supplements in the United States. By increasing circulation to the brain, ginkgo improves age-related memory problems. This is one case in which you definitely want to buy a standardized extract, because a simple whole-herb preparation could not contain enough active compounds to do any good. It takes fifty pounds of leaves from the ginkgo tree to make one pound of useful extract.

Even if your brain is working well in terms of intellect and memory, you can still be miserable and ineffective in your daily life.

Even if your brain is working well in terms of intellect and memory, you can still be miserable and ineffective in your daily life. Millions of Americans suffer from some degree of depression. The conventional medical prescriptions for depression—Prozac and Zoloft, to name a couple of the most popular—are expensive and often have disagreeable side effects. Fortunately, the plant world offers a natural alternative, St. John's wort. This common weedy plant, which has become a media star over the past year, is widely prescribed for mild depression in Europe, and has been subjected to many encouraging clinical studies.

Herbs for helping prevent more serious problems

Bilberry	Arteriosclerosis, hemorrhoids, poor night vision
Cranberry	Urinary tract infection
Ephedra	Asthma
Evening primrose oil	Essential fatty acid deficiencies
Feverfew	Migraines
Garlic	Arteriosclerosis, high cholesterol, high blood pressure
Ginkgo biloba	Memory, tinnitus, macular degeneration
Hawthorn	Angina pectoris, congestive heart failure
Licorice	Ulcers
Milk thistle	Liver problems
Saw palmetto	Benign prostatic hyperplasia
St John's wort	Mild depression

If you're taking a chemical antidepressant, you don't want to make an abrupt transition to St. John's wort, and you don't want to change at all without consulting your health-care provider. Clinical depression is nothing to play around with. But hundreds of thousands of people are finding that St. John's wort evens out the lows of mild depression. It takes at least four to six weeks of continuous use to feel the effects of this herb, and the benefits stop if you stop taking it. Again, a standardized extract will give the most reliable results.

Chapter 10: Herbal Supplements for Women

Men's and women's bodies are different, and there are herbs suited for the unique needs of each. In fact, many herbs are especially beneficial for the special conditions associated with women's reproductive health, from the onset of puberty through menopause. Since I'm not a woman, I can't write about this subject from a personal perspective as I have in other parts of this book. But I've read and researched enough to know that there are some very good herbal alternatives for the special health concerns that women deal with.

> **Many herbs are especially beneficial for the special conditions associated with women's reproductive health, from the onset of puberty through menopause.**

Menstruation, PMS, and menopause

The hormones that women's bodies produce to regulate ovulation and menstruation result in the wonders of childbirth for some women, but they also can create havoc on a monthly basis. The cramps and bloating that often accompany menstruation, the irritability and mood swings that precede it, and the profound body changes that begin to occur when menstruation ceases—all can benefit from herbal approaches that may be wiser or more effective than the synthetic hormones, tranquilizers, and pain relievers often prescribed by medical doctors.

Women's herbs tend to overlap in categories that are useful for all three conditions. Muscle relaxants such as cramp bark, and general relaxants such as valerian, kava-kava, and passion-

Herbs to Avoid During Pregnancy

Barberry
Black cohosh
Black walnut hulls
Blueberry
Blue cohosh
Catnip
Chaparral
Dong quai
Ephedra
Goldenseal
Juniper berry
Licorice
Lobelia
Motherwort
Myrrh
Osha
Pennyroyal
Pleurisy root
Shepherd's purse
Turmeric
Uva ursi
Vitex
Yarrow

Flower can ease painful cramping. These general relaxants, and a more specific mood balancer such as St. John's wort, can temper the mood swings of PMS, while vitex and black cohosh help rebalance hormones and tonify uterus. Add dong quai and Siberian ginseng to vitex

Herbs to Avoid When Breast Feeding
Black Cohosh
Ephedra

and black cohosh, and you have a powerful quartet of herbal supporters for that time of life when the body begins to shut down estrogen production. The same mood- and muscle-relaxants that have been useful previously also help with the throes of menopause. And while you may think of them more as food than herb, soy products (beans, tofu, tempeh) have the ability to mimic estrogen in the body and thus greatly ease the physical changes of menopause.

Let's look at the records of these women's herbs. Vitex has been well-researched in Europe; in controlled studies, more than 90 percent of women reported some relief of their PMS symptoms after using it. Dong quai, a species of angelica, has been used in China for thousands of years for women's health. It reduces inflammation and pain and normalizes uterine contractions—which is why pregnant women shouldn't take it. Black cohosh is native to North America, and was actually listed in the U.S. Pharmacopoeia until 1926. This is one of many good illustrations of how modern medicine has moved far away from the useful traditions to which more and more people are now returning.

Osteoporosis

As people age, changing hormonal makeup often means serious bone loss, or osteoporosis. More women than men suffer from this problem, and the cost of treating it exceeds $6 billion a year—not to mention the loss of quality of life in those who are most affected. Weight-bearing exercise and plenty of dietary calcium are what the medical community recommends. Dandelion leaf is extremely rich in calcium, and the soy products mentioned above are also loaded with calcium. Adding these to the diet, either as whole foods or supplements, can be very beneficial.

Urinary tract infections

Because of their physiology—the close

proximity of vagina, urethra, and anus, and the short distance from the urethra to the bladder—women often suffer from urinary tract infections.

Cranberry not only treats but helps prevent urinary tract infections.

Cranberry is a widely accepted treatment for avoiding infections, and its use in turn sidesteps the problem of antibiotic overuse.

The natural acids in cranberry juice discourage the growth of bacteria in the urinary tract, and they also help prevent bacteria from attaching to the bladder wall. So cranberry not only treats but prevents urinary tract infections. Commercial cranberry juice generally contains a lot of sugar, which creates its own problems. So you may prefer to consider some of the highly concentrated cranberry herbal supplements available as capsules.

Skin care

I will risk sounding sexist here by including in this chapter herbs that contribute to healthy skin.

Skin is every bit as important an organ in men as it is in women, but it's been my observation that women tend to care more about keeping their skin healthy and looking young.

Herbs such as calendula, aloe, chamomile, and others are turning up in more and more salves and lotions for the skin, as well as other cosmetic products. If you want to try these, just be careful to read the labels closely. I've often found that there's very little of the actual herb in these preparations. Be wary of those that use the name of an herb on the label just to hype the product.

Women now make up the majority of the population in our country and as the baby-boomer generation ages, more emphasis will be put on products targeted for the women of this generation. Natural, organic, and herbal products specifically designed to appeal to affluent customers will be featured. So

Be wary of products that use the name of an herb on the label just to hype the product

Herbs for improving women's health	
Black cohosh	This herb is approved by doctors in Germany for the treatment of all PMS and menopausal symptoms including hot flashes
Calendula	Dry, aging skin
Cranberry	Research indicates that this herb is effective for urinary infections.
Dandelion	Diuretic
Dong quai	The primary herb recommended in China for relief of PMS symptoms. Pregnant or nursing women should not use dong quai.
Vitex	Another excellent herb for the alleviation of PMS symptoms. Vitex may be taken with confidence because it has been extensively researched.

learn as much as you can and don't be fooled by exotic herbal names on expensive products that truly have no added value.

Chapter 11: Herbal Supplements for Men

This chapter is easier for me to write than the last one was. As a 49-year-old man, I've faced a lot of the stress-related illnesses associated with building a career, and now I'm beginning to experience other symptoms associated with aging. On top of that, I hate going to a doctor at any time, for any reason. I know a lot of other men who feel the same. So it's really encouraging to know that some herbal treatments can help me maintain energy and good health. I've already had good success with a few.

Coping with stress

When I was younger, stress-related conditions such as high blood pressure, ulcers, heart attacks, and stroke were considered men's problems. With more and more women taking high-profile positions in the workplace, juggling career and family, this is no longer the case. But I'm making special mention of these problems in this chapter because men do worry about them, and men's mortality rate is still higher than women's—for many of these stress-related reasons.

I've mentioned it in previous chapters, but it bears repeating. Garlic is a wonderful tonic herb that can be taken daily to alleviate many stress-related symptoms. I've personally gotten my blood pressure down from alarming levels to fairly normal ones with a daily garlic supplement. I eat a lot of fresh garlic, but I also take a garlic capsule every morning. Its enteric coating guarantees that the garlic won't be digested before it gets to my large intestine—where it will do the most good—and my coworkers at the office appreciate the "hidden benefits" of this form. Garlic is also very effective for reducing cholesterol.

Ulcers are a serious stress-related disease, again one that has traditionally been considered a men's problem. German research has shown that licorice (the herb, not the candy) is effective in relieving irritated stomach tissues.

Men can be just as troubled by insomnia as women, especially when life stresses are high. And the same herbs can be helpful. I've had good luck with valerian taken thirty or forty-five minutes before bed. Kava-kava and passionflower are also useful for relaxing and getting a better night's rest.

Avoiding the digital exam

As a man's level of testosterone changes, his hair starts thinning and his prostate starts enlarging. The hair problem involves acceptance (or transplants), but the prostate problem can really become annoying. It's not life-threatening, but it affects the vast majority of men over the age of 40.

A close relative of mine has a severe case of benign prostatic hyperplasia (BPH). He gets up four or five times a night to urinate, which means neither he nor his wife can get a good night's sleep. Left untreated, BPH can be painful and even result in impotence. Fortunately, there's a very effective herbal remedy for this condition.

Saw palmetto has been proven through numerous clinical trials to reduce the size of the prostate and return normal functioning to most men. This wonderful herb is inexpensive, effective, and produces no side effects when taken as directed. However, I will say this: If you're having problems with your prostate, you *must* bite the bullet and see a doctor to rule out anything more serious than BPH.

Another herb that has also been proven effective for BPH is pygeum. You'll often find new men's products that combine saw palmetto and pygeum. I'm currently taking a standardized extract of saw palmetto every day as a preventive measure. It can't hurt, and as far as I know, it's helping.

Diminished sex drive

Recently, the media has been full of reports about the new anti-impotence drug, Viagra. It's gotten some glowing reviews, but it's very expensive and has some potentially serious side effect—including death! Before trying Viagra myself, I would try Chinese ginseng. It's been used in the Orient for centuries as a general restorative, and it may increase a man's sex drive.

Herbs for Improving Men's Health	
Garlic	Combats high blood pressure and high cholesterol
Ginseng	Boosts energy, serves as tonic
Hawthorn	Helps regulate the heart
Hops	Eases insomnia
Kava-kava	Soothes anxiety
Pygeum	Helps regulate prostate gland
Saw palmetto	Helps regulate prostate gland
Tea tree	Fights skin fungus

Chapter 12: Up-and-Coming Herbs

I t's exciting to see new herbal products being introduced in this country. As traditional Chinese medicine (TCM) and Indian ayurvedic medicine become better known, the herbs recommended by these systems are finding their way into Western use. Medicinal herbs are generally regarded more seriously in Asia and Europe, and are often prescribed alongside western-style pharmaceuticals. So the research from those parts of the world tends to be abundant and rigorous. Outstanding research has been done in Europe and Asia and some of their tried and tested herbs are now being introduced in the United States. Botanical exploration is also being conducted in the endangered tropical rain forests of the world, and at least a small portion of the rich biodiversity of those regions is beginning to be looked at in terms of its medicinal promise.

Here are a few relatively recent entries into the U.S. market. Some are already in widespread use, others you will likely hear more about over the next years.

Bitter gourd (*Mormordica charantia*). Cultivated throughout India for its fruit, and used there for a host of ailments, bitter gourd is currently being studied for its ability to regulate blood sugar levels and help with diabetes. It is toxic unless properly processed.

> **Medicinal herbs are generally regarded more seriously in Asia and Europe, and are often prescribed alongside western-style pharmaceuticals.**

Black cohosh (*Cimicifuga racemosa*). One of the herbs mentioned in Chapter 10 as a treatment for menopausal symptoms, black cohosh is widely used in Europe and gaining popularity in this country. Like echinacea, it's native to North America. It is currently being overharvested, which may affect future price and availability.

Cat's claw *(Uncaria tomentosa).* A rainforest herb that has gained popularity for its reputation for supporting and stimulating the immune system. The standardized supplement has been the subject of recent research and preliminary results show a possible anti-tumor effect.

Horse chestnut (*Aesculus hippocastanum)*. If you ever had horse-chestnut-burr fights when you were a kid, it will probably seem strange to think of any part of this fine hardwood tree as a medicinal herb. But standardized extracts are now being offered, and European research shows horse chestnut to be especially effective for increasing circulation and reducing varicose veins and general swelling in the legs. The *"horse"* in its name, incidentally, refers to its traditional use for treating respiratory problems in horses.

Kava-kava (*Piper mythysticum*). This herb has been used in the islands of the South Pacific for centuries, and it's been widely available in this country for a couple of years. Now, media attention is beginning to make it a household word. Kava-kava soothes anxiety and stress, relaxing muscles and reducing tension while allowing one to think clearly. And when taken at appropriate dosages, it has no negative side effects. As it has gained in popularity, it has gotten to be in short supply.

St. John's wort (*Hypericum perforatum*) This herb

has been used for centuries to treat a variety of problems and it is one of the leading herbs prescribed by European physicians for the treatment of depression. It's been around in this country for quite some time, too, but has become extremely popular since the fall of 1997 when a major television news program gave it high marks. Supply is only now beginning to catch up with demand after this media exposure.

Turmeric (*Curcuma longa*). Another Indian medicinal herb that has been common in this country as a kitchen spice for generations, turmeric is now regarded as a strong antioxidant. It also contains a compound that works to reduce swelling and inflammation.

Maitake (*Grifola frondosa*). This medicinal mushroom has been used to reduce high blood pressure and protect the liver. Early research indicates that it may inhibit tumor growth as well.

Reishi (*Ganoderma lucidum*). This mushroom has been revered in China as a general tonic because it relieves a number of health problems and restores wellness. Reishi is gaining popularity in the United States as it becomes more available.

New combination herbal products

In Traditional Chinese Medicine—in most traditional herbal medicine, in fact—most remedies are combinations rather than single herbs. Intuition and empirical evidence have pointed to synergies that may exist among herbs. In the United States, early herbalists made combinations, and most practicing herbalists still do. But if you look at the commercially-available herbal products in this country, single-herb preparations far outsell combination products. This could change. Currently being developed by some of the major manufacturers are new combination products that add vitamins, minerals, and other nutritional substances to herbs.

For example, one new product for the heart contains hawthorn, Coenzyme Q 10, vitamin E, and folic acid. These nutrients have all been proven good for the heart and for circulation. If this kind of combination product becomes a trend, as it appears to be doing, consumers will benefit because combinations are cheaper than buying separate supplements.

And finally

New herbal products are being developed and introduced each month. More and more people are turning to herbs, and more and more stores are selling them. This rapid growth and ever-changing market creates even more confusion in making choices. I highly recommend that you find a reliable source for buying your herbs and good brands you trust and then stick with them.

You'll find a reference section on page 113 that lists sources you can turn to for more information. Use it with confidence when you have additional questions about herbal supplements.

I know that taking herbal supplements has enhanced my health and well being. I hope you will enjoy the same benefits I have and that this book will help you make good choices. I wish you a long and healthy life.

USING HERBAL ALTERNATIVES

DR. JAMES A. DUKE

Make sure of the diagnosis. Self-diagnosis is a risky business, and best left to well-trained physicians. Once you're confident of a diagnosis, though, then discuss with your physician how to treat it: drugs, herbs, some combination of the two, or any of the foregoing plus diet, exercise, and lifestyle changes.

Watch out for side effects. If you have an unpleasant reaction to an herb, such as dizziness, nausea, or headache, cut back on your dosage or stop taking the herb. Listen to your body. If the herb doesn't feel right, don't take it.

Beware of interactions. Pharmaceutical medications sometimes interact badly with each other and with certain foods. The same goes for herbal medicines. Always be particularly careful when taking more than one drug or herb or a combination of a drug and herb. If you suspect a bad interaction, consult your physician or pharmacist.

If you're pregnant, take special precautions. As a general rule, you shouldn't take herbs while you're pregnant unless you discuss your selections with your obstetrician, because quite a few herbs can increase the risk of miscarriage.

With these thoughts in mind, use the following chart for your good health. Share it with your health care provider, and use it to learn more. Ample research exists to guide you safely and healthfully to taking care of your body by using alternatives to the pharmaceuticals our society so readily turns to.

HERBAL SUBSTITUTES FOR COMMON PHARMACEUTICALS

JAMES A. DUKE PH.D.

Ailment	Commonly Prescribed Pharmaceutical	Herbal Option
Acne	Retin-A, Tetracycline	Tea Tree (external); Calendula
Allergies	Synthetic Antihistamines	Garlic, Stinging Nettle, Ginkgo
Anxiety	Ativan, Xanax, Klonopin	Hops, Kava-kava, Valerian
Arthritic Pain	Tylenol, other NSAIDS*	Cayenne (external); Celery Seed, Ginger, Turmeric
Athlete's Foot	Griseofulvin	Tea Tree (external); Garlic
Boils	Erythromycin	Tea Tree, Slippery Elm (both external)
BPH (Benign Prostatic Hyperplasia)	Hytrin, Proscar	Saw Palmetto, Evening Primrose
Body Odor, Perspiration	Commercial Deodorants, Antiperspirants	Coriander, Sage
Bronchitis	Atropine	Echinacea, Garlic
Bruises	Analgesics	Arnica, St. John's wort, Yarrow, Plantain (all external)

Ailment	Commonly Prescribed Pharmaceutical	Herbal Option
Burns	Silvadene Cream	Aloe (external)
Colds	Decongestants	Echinacea, Ginger, Lemon Balm, Garlic
Constipation	Laxatives	Flaxseed, Psyllium
Cuts, Scrapes, Abscesses	Topical Antibiotics	Tea Tree, Calendula, Plantain (all external)
Mild Depression	Prozac, Elavil, Trazodone, Zoloft	St. John's wort
Diarrhea	Imodium, Lomotil	Bilberry, Raspberry
Dysmenorrhea (painful menstruation)	Naprosyn	Kava-kava, Raspberry
Earache	Antibiotics	Echinacea, Garlic, Mullein
Eczema (itchy rash)	Corticosteroids	Chamomile
Atopic Eczema (allergy-related rash)	Corticosteroids, Sedatives, Antihistamines	Evening Primrose
Flu	Tylenol	Echinacea, Elderberry

Herbal substitutes for common pharmaceuticals

Ailment	Commonly Prescribed Pharmaceutical	Herbal Option
Gas	Mylanta, Gaviscon, Simethicone	Dill, Fennel, Peppermint
Gingivitis (gum inflammation)	Peridex	Chamomile, Echinacea, Sage
Halitosis (bad breath)	Listerine	Cardamom, Parsley, Peppermint
Hay Fever	Antihistamines, Decongestants	Stinging Nettle
Headache	Aspirin, other NSAIDs*	Peppermint (external); Feverfew, Willow
Heartburn	Pepto-Bismol, Tums	Angelica, Chamomile, Peppermint
Hemorrhoids	Tucks	Plantain, Witch Hazel (both external)
Hepatitis	Interferon	Dandelion, Milk Thistle, Turmeric
Herpes	Acyclovir	Lemon Balm
High Cholesterol	Mevacor	Garlic
Hives	Benadryl	Stinging Nettle

Ailment	Commonly Prescribed Pharmaceutical	Herbal Option
Indigestion	Antacids, Reglan	Chamomile, Ginger, Peppermint
Insomnia	Halcion, Ativan	Chamomile, Hops, Lemon Balm, Valerian, Kava-kava, Evening Primrose
Irregularity	Metamucil	Flaxseed, Plantain, Senna
Low Back Pain	Aspirin, Analgesics	Cayenne (external); Thyme
Male Pattern Baldness	Rogaine	Saw Palmetto
Migraine	Cafergot, Sumatriptan, Verapamil	Feverfew
Motion Sickness	Dramamine	Ginger
Nail Fungus	Ketoconazole	Tea Tree (external)
Night Blindness	Vitamin A	Bilberry
PMS	NSAIDs*, Diuretics, Analgesics	Chaste Tree, Evening Primrose

Herbal substitutes for common pharmaceuticals

Ailment	Commonly Prescribed Pharmaceutical	Herbal Option
Rhinitis (nasal inflammation)	Cromolyn, Vancenase	Echinacea
Shingles	Acyclovir	Cayenne (external); Lemon Balm
Sprain	NSAIDs*	Arnica, Calendula
Stress	Diazepam	Kava-kava, Valerian
Tinnitus (ringing in the ears)	Steroids	Ginkgo
Toothache	NSAIDs*	Cloves, Willow
Urinary Tract Infections	Sulfa Drugs	Cranberry, Stinging Nettle
Vaginitis	Clindamycin, Flagyl	Garlic, Goldenseal

*NSAIDs are nonsteroidal anti-inflammatory drugs

Reprinted from *Herbs for Health* magazine, Nov/Dec 1997, with permission.

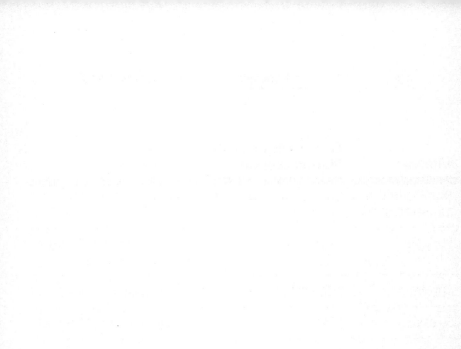

ADDITIONAL READING

Books

Balch, James F. and Phyllis A. Balch. *Prescription for Nutritional Healing*. New York: Avery Publishing Group, Inc., 1990.

Carper, Jean. *The Food Pharmacy: Dramatic New Evidence That Food Is Your Best Medicine*. New York: Bantam Books, 1988.

DeSilva, Derrick M. *Ask the Doctor: Herbs & Supplements for Better Health*. Loveland: Interweave Press, 1997.

Duke, James A. *The Green Pharmacy: New Discoveries in Herbal Remedies for Common Diseases and Conditions from the World's Foremost Authority on Healing Herbs*. Emmaus: Rodale Press, Inc., 1997.

Foster, Steven. *Herbs for Your Health: A handy guide for knowing and using 50 common herbs*. Loveland: Interweave Press, 1996.

_____. *101 Medicinal Herbs: An Illustrated Guide*. Loveland: Interweave Press, 1998.

Gagnon, Daniel. *Liquid Herbal Drops In Everyday Use.* Santa Fe: Botanical Research and Education Institute, 1996.

Hobbs, Christopher. *Echinacea: The Immune Herb.* Loveland: Botanica Press/Interweave Press, 1990.

_____. *Ginkgo: Elixir of Youth.* Loveland: Botanica Press/Interweave Press, 1991.

_____. *The Ginsengs: A User's Guide.* Loveland: Botanica Press/Interweave Press, 1996.

_____ and Stephen Brown. *Saw Palmetto: The Herb for Prostate Health.* Loveland: Botanica Press/Interweave Press, 1997.

_____. *Stress and Natural Healing.* Loveland: Botanica Press/Interweave Press, 1997.

_____. *St. John's Wort: The Mood Enhancing Herb.* Loveland: Botanica Press/Interweave Press, 1997.

_____ and Kathi Keville. *Women's Herbs, Women's Health*. Loveland: Botanica Press/Interweave Press, 1998.

Keville, Kathi. *Herbs for Health and Healing*. Emmaus: Rodale Press, Inc., 1996.

Kowalchik, Claire and Judith Benn Hurley, eds. *Rodale's Illustrated Encyclopedia of Herbs*. Emmaus: Rodale Press, Inc., 1987.

Mindell, Earl. *Earl Mindell's Herb Bible*. New York: Simon & Schuster, 1992.

_____. *Dr. Earl Mindell's What You Should Know About Herbs for Your Health*. New Canaan: Keats Publishing, Inc., 1996.

Tyler, Varro E. *Herbs of Choice: The Therapeutic Use of Phytomedicinals*. New York: Pharmaceutical Products Press, 1994.

Weil, Andrew. *Spontaneous Healing*. New York: Alfred A. Knopf, 1995.

Periodicals

Anderson, L.A. "Concern Regarding Herbal Toxicities: Case reports and counseling Tips," *The Annals of Pharmacotherapy*, January, 1996, Vol. 30, pp. 79-80.

Brown, D. "Ginkgo Biloba Extract for Age-Related Cognitive Decline and Early-Stage Dementia Clinical Overview," *Quarterly Review of Natural Medicine*. Summer, 1997, pp. 91-96.

Chan, Thomas Y. K. and Julian A. J. H. Critchley. "Usage and Adverse Effects of Chinese Herbal Medicines," *Human and Experimental Toxicology*, 1996, No. 15, pp. 5-12.

Hochswender, Cynthia. "The Big Nine: An Expert's Guide to Growing and Using the Most Healthful Herbs," *American Health*, June 1997, pp. 74-77.

Hooper, Joseph. "Back to Nature: A Guided Trip Down the Aisles of the Hormone and Herb

Supplement Supermarket," *Men's Journal*, March, 1997, pp. 87-89 & 91.

Muir, Maya. "Mint, Rue, and Rattlesnake Meat," *Alternative & Complementary Therapies*, November/December, 1996, pp. 366-372.

Upton, Roy, ed. "St. John's Wort Hypericum perforatum Monograph," *HerbalGram*, Summer, 1997, No. 40, pp. 1-32.

Other

Blumenthal, Mark. "Therapeutic Monographs," *Popular Herbs in the U.S. Market*, pp. 1-66.

National Institutes of Health. "NIH Statement on Hypericum," 1997.

Nutrition Business Journal, September, 1996, Vol. I, No. 2.

Nutrition Business Journal, April, 1997, Vol. II, No. 4.

Resources for Additional Information

American Botanical Council
PO Box 201660
Austin, TX 78720
512/331-8868
e-mail abc@herbalgram.org
www.herbalgram.org

American Association of Naturopathic Physicians
2366 Eastlake Avenue E Suite 322
Seattle, WA 98102
206/298-0126
www.naturopathic.org

The American Association of Oriental Medicine
433 Front Street
Catasauqua, PA 18032
610/266-1433
e-mail aaom1@aol.com
www.aaom.org

American Herbal Products Association
4733 Bethesda Avenue Suite 345
Bethesda, MD 20814
301/951-3204
e-mail AHPA@ix.netcom.com
www.ahpa.org

American Herbalist Guild
PO Box 70
Roosevelt, UT 84066
435/722-8434
e-mail ahgoffice@earthlink.net
www.earthlink.net

Health Net Online
www.Healthnet.com

Herb Research Foundation
1007 Pearl Street Suite 200
Boulder, CO 80302
303/449-2265
e-mail info@herbs.org
www.herbs.org

National Nutritional Foods Association
3931 MacArthur Boulevard Suite 101
Newport Beach, CA 92660
714/622-6272
e-mail NNFA@aol.com
www.nnfa.org

The Natural Healthcare Hotline
(for consumers, part of Herb Research
Foundation, funded by members)
800/226-4611

The School of Phytotherapy
10401 Montgomery Parkway NE
Albuquerque, NM 87111
505/275-0620
e-mail phyto@swcp.com

The School of Natural Healing
PO Box 412
Springville, VT 84663
1-800-372-8255

INDEX